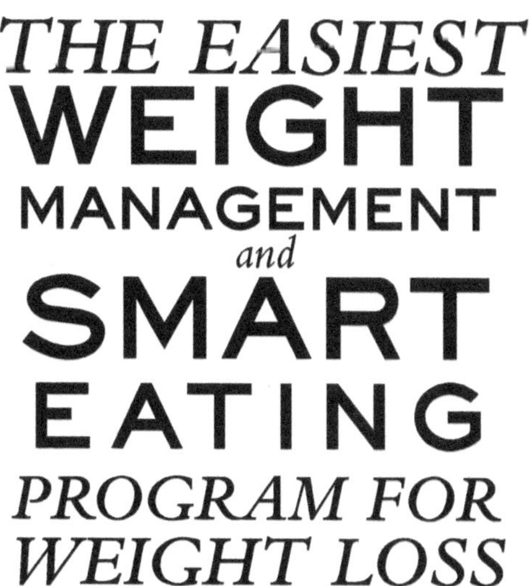

THE EASIEST WEIGHT MANAGEMENT and SMART EATING PROGRAM FOR WEIGHT LOSS

Philip Hamrick

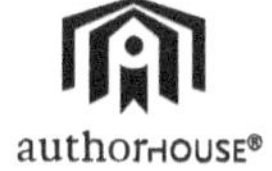

authorHOUSE®

AuthorHouse™
1663 Liberty Drive
Bloomington, IN 47403
www.authorhouse.com
Phone: 1-800-839-8640

Published by AuthorHouse 1/29/2013

ISBN: 978-1-4817-0964-4 (sc)
ISBN: 978-1-4817-0963-7 (e)

Library of Congress Control Number: 2013901142

Table of Contents

Introduction

With the obesity problem in this county, this book is being written to help and inspire everyone that is trying to lose weight and to keep it off, or if you need to gain weight, by sharing my techniques, smart eating habits and weight management program I personally learned and used myself to lose 220 pounds that can easily be used by everyone no matter how much weight you need to lose and that and can be used by males, females, young and old. A new study suggests that by 2030 nearly half of all Americans will be obese which would mean millions of dollars more for the diet industry. Obesity is also a cause of a lot of our health problems in this country. Belly fat increases the risk of developing diabetes, heart disease, high blood fats, hypertension, stroke, sleep apnea, arthritis and some cancers. Eating habits are learned at a young age, as we get older, our eating habits get worse. Foods become an obsession, we eat just to be eating and it sometimes makes us feel good. Instead of eating because we are hungry, or to survive, we're eating to just be eating. I'm not a doctor or a nutrition expert, but have done some research into this matter and have personal experience pertaining to my own weight loss and weight management program. The word diet means temporary and failure, most of my friends, including myself have tried numerous diets, some worked with limited results, and some didn't, but after coming off the diet I always gained the weight back plus more. I didn't learn smart eating habits or weight management during my dieting. It seems the diet industry is always putting out a new diet pill or fade in the hopes that we will buy into it, and a lot of people do, with promises of easy weight loss without having to do any diet or exercise. Our society is now being bought up to expect everything to be given without having to work for it. I just read an ad for a weight loss product. Clinically proven, weight loss that works, not a diet, no food restrictions, no counting calories, no prepackaged meals to buy, no exercise required, but in small letters at the bottom of the ad said for best results for weight loss using this product was by using their sensible diet and exercise program along with their product. After buying their product, you still have to pay to join their online service to obtain their diet and exercise program or you have to buy extra videos. Save your money, learn smart eating habits and spend your money on something else. None of these weight loss products or fads diets work without doing a diet plan and exercise program, but the problem is after most people lose the weight, if they lost any at all, they gained it back because they hadn't learned smart eating habits to keep the weight off.

Common signs you're looking at a fad diet:

> The diet claims fast and easy weight loss without having to do any diet or exercise.
>
> The diet requires you to eliminate certain food or bad food groups. Some people do need to eliminate certain foods due to allergies or metabolic disorders, but most people need to choose a variety of foods from all the food groups every day to include proteins, good (non-sugar) carbohydrates and fats, but in limited portions.
>
> The diet requires you to include dietary supplements labeled as fat burners and metabolism boosters. Read

> the ad closely, you will see a disclaimer in tiny letters at the bottom of most ads.
>
> The diet requires you to eat a combination of required foods for results, stating that your body can't digest carbohydrates with proteins or fats. Your digestive system uses different enzymes for digestion of different foods and they cancel each other out, they all work together. You just have to eat small portions of each food group but only limiting your intake of fats and sugars.

Fad diets may be effective for weight loss in the short term because you will lose some extra fluid as well as some fat. The weight loss is usually temporary because when you complete your diet chances are you'll return to your old eating habits, and in time, your weight will be right back where it was before starting your diet. There are two problems with diet fades. One, you will never develop good smart eating habits, and after you discontinue the diet there is a great chance you will gain all the weight back, plus more because you would be accustomed to eating without any regard to the consequences. Two, though you would be losing weight, the diet would be taking its toll on your overall health.

There are some good diet plans available, but there costly. Look for diet plans that offer you good eating habits that will includes all the food groups, and also encourages you to increase your activity levels. Also a few plans actually provide you with pre-packaged food items containing nutritional information and calorie counts. But when you complete your diet plan you should have learned smart eating habits to keep the weight off you had lost, plus be able to manage your weight the rest of your life. You can never return to your old bad eating habits because you will gain your weight back.

Hopefully this book will help you to learn smart eating habits and a weight management program.

Losing weight is fairly simple, I did it. It's a matter of burning more calories than you take in, by cutting down on your calories you eat daily, or adding more activities to your daily routine and sometime you may have to do both. Hopefully this book and techniques will help you like it helped me in losing weight and being able to keep it off, I was able to lose 220 pounds and now I am using the techniques in this book to keep the weight off.

Disclaimer

This book was written about my own experience dealing with my own Weight Management Program, Weight Loss and Weight Control, and to share the information and techniques I learned and used throughout the years with anyone this information may help. Information in this book should not be used as a substitute for any type of personal medical advice. Before starting any diet or exercise program you should consult your doctor, mostly if you have any type of medical condition or are on any medications.

Chapter I
History

I was born in 1952 a large baby 8lbs plus, I was overweight my whole life. I always thought I was born fat and would die fat. In my early years I was taught bad eating habits. I was told to be a football player I had to eat, but I wasn't taught my weight had to match my height. I was considered chubby up and through the 8th grade, I was always considered by the weight chart as being 30 pounds overweight. In the 9th grade I discovered barbells, and started a weight training program (lifting weights and a diet program), which in those days wasn't popular yet. I was able to turn the 30 pounds of overweight fat to lean muscle. I was able to maintain this up through high school at around 200 pounds. I was 5 ft. 9 in. tall and according to the height and weight chart I should have weighed 168 pounds. In my twenty's I wanted to increase my lifts, but I didn't want to use any drugs or supplements, so I just ate well. My weight jumped up to 230 pounds but was lean and a good weight, and at that weight I could bench press 460 pounds. In my late twenty's I got lazy and stopped my weight training program, but did nothing to curb my bad eating habits. I continued eating as if I was still exercising, I gained another 40 pounds and in my thirty's I maintained a weight of around 280 pounds, but my lean muscle mass had disappeared. On and off I'd try different diet fads, sometimes I'd lose weight and sometimes I wouldn't. If I lost weight, as soon as I would get to a certain weight I'd come off the diet and gain all the weight back plus more. My biggest problem was that I just liked to eat, I loved food. In my forty's my weight had ballooned to around a weight of 330 pounds. Twice I started exercising and dieting and lost 100 pounds each time, but always returned to non-exercising and keeping bad eating habits. At 57 my weight had exceeded 425 pounds. My blood pressure was out of sight 155/115, my knees were giving out, and I couldn't run more than 10 yards without getting out of breath. I did research on the internet, and using past history and personal experience and techniques I had learned and used, I put a program together to eat whatever I wanted within reason and to lose 220 pounds and to keep it off doing it the natural way without diet fads, pills, or operations, at no extra cost except a dedication to a life change I must do the rest of my life with smart eating habits and a good weight management program.

In the beginning of my weight loss I would avoid the elementary school playground my waist line was probably a 68. The kids would see me going by and scream out and call me pig man. Kids are cruel, so I tried to avoid the area when they were out on recess and would take another route until I got my weight down to where I didn't look that bad.

A group of senior citizens from the center I would walk past every morning now gets out and walks every morning claiming I inspired them to get up and out which is my private group that has supported me the whole way.

During my weight loss, I had a town watch me disappear little at a time going from 425 pounds to 200 pounds. When I'm out walking or running now I have numerous people stopping me all the time complimenting me on my weight loss and health changes, and telling me how I also inspired them to get out and start exercising themselves. This made me feel good even though I didn't mean to inspire anyone, but I was glad that I was able to inspire someone else to get out and help them to better themselves.

CHAPTER 2

Calorie Components

In order to understand weight management and weight control you must understand the three components that makeup a calorie and how these components are an important part of everyone's daily diet.

Protein

What is a protein, and why is it essential. Webster's Dictionary defines a protein as a very large group of highly complex nitrogenous compounds occurring in living matter and composed of amino acids which are essential for tissue repair and growth. Proteins build and repair muscles, and are the basis of our body's organs, hormones, enzymes, and antibodies to fight infection. Proteins are also an emergency fuel for our bodies in the absence of sufficient carbohydrates and fats. This is why weight loss should be gradual so to preserve protein levels in muscles and other body organs. In addition to keeping hunger in check, regular doses of protein help to keep body composition, (the amount of fat relative to muscle), in better proportion. Along with calcium and vitamin D, protein helps you to preserve muscle mass as you drop pounds. Proteins are found in almost every food product.

Fats

Fats in food are a mixture of 3 basic types, saturated,

monounsaturated, and polyunsaturated. Animal fats found mainly in full cream milks, cheeses, butters, creams, fatty meats and processed foods are considered saturated fats while plant oils and fish oils are mainly monounsaturated and polyunsaturated fats. Trans fats come from hydrogenated vegetable oils and shortenings which is common in commercial baked and fried food products.

Carbohydrates

Carbohydrates are essential to good health. They are the main source of fuel for the body. The non-sugar item carbohydrates provide important vitamins, minerals, antioxidants and fiber which helps protect against heart disease, diabetes, hypertension, constipation and many other diseases and also helps the body produce serotonin, a brain chemical that helps control appetite and overeating. Carbohydrates can be found in different forms of food such as sugar items, and the non-sugar items are fruits, vegetables, milk, and starches in whole grains, legumes, nuts, and seeds.

Calorie

What is a calorie, and why is it important to know what a calorie has to do with weight gains and loss or maintaining your weight. Webster's Dictionary defines calorie as a measurement of the amount of heat or energy produced by food. Calories in food are derived from a combination of proteins, fats and carbohydrates that make up the food product. Fats in food have over double the calories than proteins and carbohydrates found in food, so the higher the fat content of the food, the higher the calories in that food product would be. It takes 3,500 calories to equal one pound of weight.

Chapter 3

Weight Management

Weight management is managing to keep your current weight at a reasonable constant weight. This can be achieved when the number of calories that you eat is equal to the number of calories your body uses. The most sensible way to lose weight and manage your body weight for life is by eating smart and adding more activities to your daily routines, and if possible by exercising more. I implemented a plan I could live with that worked for me. I ate what I wanted which included home cooking, restaurants, fast food, parties and special events not restricting myself to any particular food group. Your body burns so many calories a day just for normal body functions which is your Basal Metabolic Rate (BMR), and adding your daily activities gives you the total calories needed to maintain a certain body weight which is known as your Active Metabolic Rate (AMR), which is your metabolism. Metabolism is the process your body uses to break down food. If your calorie intake matches your daily AMR you will maintain that body weight. If your calorie intake exceeded your daily AMR then you will gain weight which is stored in your body fat, for every 3,500 calories stored you will gain one pound. If your calorie intake is less than your daily AMR then you will lose weight from stored fat taken from your body fat, for every 3,500 calories taken from your body fat you will lose one pound. If you want to lose weight you need to decrease your calorie intake during the day by eating less or increase your physical activity, or both. If you were to reduce your current calorie intake by 500 calories every day, you would lose about one pound each week. Also don't waste time on a crash diet, this would be dropping your daily intake calories way below your daily calories needed each day. When you go on a crash diet your metabolism slows down thinking its starving and you will burn fewer calories than normal or your body stores everything you do eat as fat, defeating the purpose of trying to lose weight. Always eat at least three regular portion size meals a day, or five small portion size meals a day. It is recommended to eat five small portion size meals a day. This will keep your metabolism up and will increase your energy level and AMR throughout the day.

Review and recommended tips to boost your AMR which will help you burn more calories:

> Exercise will help your body burn more calories efficiently, especially if you hit the gym. By strength training a couple times a week you'll increase your metabolism from slowing down and burn more calories. Not only does muscle weigh more than fat, but muscle uses more energy also. The average person that strength trains 30 to 40 minutes a day twice a week will increase their resting metabolism by 100 calories a day, even on the days they don't make it to the gym. While doing cardio, the next time you run, swim or walk, ramp up your intensity for 30 second intervals, returning to your normal speed afterwards. Experts say using this strategy will help you consume more oxygen and make your system work harder and burn more calories. Example: Start your exercise at a normal

speed, increase your speed for 30 seconds, then return to your normal speed for 30 seconds. If running or walking outside you can use markers, like telephone poles, run the length of one pole and then walk the other length. Continue this until you complete your workout.

Eating lots of fish rich in omega-3 fatty acids, like salmon, herring and tuna, helps speed up your metabolism. Omega-3s balance blood sugar, and reduces inflammation which helps to regulate your metabolism.

Drinking green tea daily, new evidence shows the active ingredient catechin may speed up your metabolism. It is suggested that catechins may improve fat oxidation and thermogenesis, which is your body's production of energy, or heat from digestion.

Don't crash diet or skip meals cutting down on your calorie intake. If you cut out too many calories your metabolism thinks it starving and puts the breaks on fat burning to conserve energy. To keep your metabolism up while dieting, eat enough calories to at least match your resting BMR.

The period after an intense workout session which is known as excess post exercise oxygen consumption (EPOC), your body can take hours to recover and return to its previous resting BMR. Your body is burning more calories than it normally would hours after you've finished your workout.

Never skip breakfast. Eating a nutrient rich morning

meal containing a balance of protein, carbohydrates and fats shortly after getting out of bed will wake up your metabolism.

Eating small meals throughout the day is a proven strategy that helps curb hunger and eating fewer calories overall. Experts are promoting nibbling versus gorging as a way to keep metabolism running by holding blood sugar levels steady and preventing insulin spikes. Enjoy five small meals a day, divide your usual day's calories by five, this will be your calories per meal.

Cut back on the Trans fats. Trans fats slow down your body's ability to burn fat. Trans fat binds to fat and liver cells and slows metabolism. Eating trans fats are not only high in calories but can also lead to insulin resistance and cripple your metabolism and cause weight gain.

Going organic and eating fruits, vegetables and grains grown without pesticides will keep your fat burning system running higher because they don't expose your thyroid to toxins.

Eat more protein. Your body digests protein slower than fats and carbohydrates, so you feel fuller longer. It may even give your metabolism a boost. In a process called thermogenesis, your body uses about 10% of its calorie intake for digestion. Because it takes longer to burn protein than carbohydrates and fats, your body expends more calories absorbing the nutrients in a high protein diet. Diets high in protein may help preserve lean body mass, which is the best fat burner of all, but also include good non-sugar carbohydrates and limit your fat intake.

Example: 3-1 Calorie Chart Results

Daily Calories Cut/Overeaten	Weekly Calories Cut/Overeaten	Weekly Weight in Pounds Loss or Gained
500	3500	1
600	4200	1.2
700	4900	1.4
800	5600	1.6
900	6300	1.8
1000	7000	2

Monthly Weight in Pounds Loss or Gained	Yearly Weight in Pounds Loss or Gained
4	48
5	60
6	72
7	84
8	96
9	108

Use the Calorie Chart Results above to see what your weight gains or losses would be on a weekly, monthly or yearly time frame by cutting or adding daily calories.

Example: 3-2 Height and Weight Chart

Height	Weight Range (Females)	Weight Range (Males)
4'7"	86	108
4'8"	88	110
4'9"	92	114
4'10"	97	120
4'11"	99	123
5'0"	101	127
5'1"	105	130
5'2"	110	136
5'3"	112	140
5'4"	114	145
5'5"	119	150
5'6"	123	156
5'7"	127	158
5'8"	129	162
5'9"	134	167
5'10"	138	173
5'11"	143	178
6'0"	145	182
6'1"	149	187
6'2"	156	193
6'3"	158	198
6'4"	162	202
6'5"	170	211
6'6"	172	215
6'7"	175	220

These are only recommended weights, the Height and Weight Chart doesn't take into consideration a person's body frame or lean muscle mass, this chart is for a small body frame with a normal lean muscle body mass. Add 10 to 20 pounds for person with a larger body frame (medium or large), or if you have a larger lean muscle body mass. Your true weight is what you feel comfortable at or what your doctor may recommend.

CHAPTER 4

Weight Management and Smart Eating Program

A weight management program is a plan that gives your body the nutrients it need every day while staying within your daily calorie goals for weight loss. A weight management program eating plan emphasizes eating a combination of lean meats, poultry, fish, fruits, vegetables, whole grains, and fat free or low fat milk and dairy products to include beans, eggs and nuts low in saturated fats, trans fat, cholesterol, sodium or added sugar and practice eating controlled portion sizes. Smart eating is the understanding of what a calorie is and how it effects weight management. Given all the tools provided you can design a weight management program you can live with the rest of your life modified to your own personnel needs as needed. Don't plan extreme goals, it's a slow process, and it's only safe to lose 1 to 2 pounds per week, depending on the amount of weight you need to lose. It shouldn't be difficult to lose weight, just cut down on your intake calories every day, and if possible increase your daily activities. Often tempting foods, stress, emotional factors, and lack of time tend to get in the way of successful weight loss and management. You need to change bad eating habits into good smart eating habits so you can reach your target weight and maintain that weight throughout your life.

The most important aspect of maintaining a weight

management and smart eating program is whether or not you can stick to it. You need to be able to eat that way for a long time to lose the weight and eat that way the rest of your life to keep the weight off that you lost. The first thing you need to consider to do is choose a weight management and smart eating program plan that is easiest for you to follow. If you don't know what plan fits you best, you can always give a plan a two week try. This way you can see how you feel and find out how easy the plan is to follow. You can also modify the plan as you go along to fit your needs, and see if your plan is too hard for you or too easy, but never go back to your old bad eating habits, and remember to use smart eating habits and choose healthy foods no matter which plan you use. Set realistic goals, it is only healthy to lose 1 or 2 pounds a week safely. The first week you may lose fluid weight which will be 5 to 10 pounds of easy weight loss, don't expect any more, then focus on 1 to 2 pound per week. If it took 10 years to gain 50 pounds, don't expect to lose that weight in 2 or 3 months. It is important to keep track of the foods you eat by writing down and keeping a diary tracking the calories that you eat each day. You can also go out on the internet and find an on line Food Diary to assist you in tracking your daily calories. It seems like everyone around you will be eating what they want and this will tempt you to go back to your old bad eating habits, but with will power and following your smart eating program this will help keep you on track to losing weight and keeping it off. There may be a day or two you may fall back to your old bad eating habits, don't beat yourself up over it, one day here or there is OK, but remember to get back on track on the next meal or day.

Here are some smart eating tips to assist you losing weight and will help to keep the weight off after you've lost it.

Review and recommended Smart Eating Tips:

Never skip meals. Skipping or missing meals can cause a dip in your blood sugar levels. This leads to the slowing down of your metabolism and energy level causing you to make bad eating choices because you are left hungry and will eat more food which will cause you to consume more calories throughout the day when you do eat. Maintaining your blood sugar and energy levels throughout the day by eating small amounts of food throughout the day will keep your metabolism and energy levels up. You might prefer eating 5 smaller meals rather than 3 large ones a day.

Leave food on your plate, the older you get, the more your metabolism slows, this will help you consume less calories. Put the extra food in a zip locked bag or sealed container and eat latter or save for another meal.

Never go on a diet when you are under stress.

You should not try to lose more than 1 to 2 pounds a week.

To lose weight for good, you must know that you can't go back to your old eating habits, this is a lifestyle change you must follow the rest of your life.

Never crash diet or eat less than the recommended calories a day, this will slow down your metabolism and your energy level.

Never grocery shop when you're hungry. This will likely make you buy bad food choices.

A slip up doesn't have to lead to an entire day of

overeating, correct this by making a better choice at your next meal.

Cut down food portions, but never cut out any categories. Use portion control and cut portions of food instead of removing entire categories such as carbohydrates and fats. Properly combine proteins, good non-sugar carbohydrates, and limit your fats to achieve a balance energy intake. A healthy diet also includes a mix of whole grains, fruits, and vegetables. Each person has individual needs based on their age, sex, physical and activity levels.

Never skip breakfast. People that eat breakfast on the averages, eats less calories throughout the day.

Eat a lot of protein early in the day. Protein digests at a slower rate than simple carbohydrates or fats, so you'll feel full longer.

Eat slowly, you'll eat less and be satisfied with eating less food and consuming fewer calories.

If you have trouble controlling the amount you eat of a favorite snack or dessert, such as ice cream, cakes and pies, do not bring it into your home, eat it only at special events.

Make your lunch at home and bring it to work. It will probably be more nutritious and contain fewer calories.

Get enough sleep, at least 6 to 8 hours a night. People who fail to get enough restorative sleep experience many hormonal shifts that influence appetite. You're more likely to give in to cravings when you're tired.

Avoid eating close to bedtime because your body will spend energy digesting the food rather than shifting into restorative sleep. Don't eat at least three hours before going to bed, if you must have something, drink a glass of milk, which may increase serotonin levels.

Eat only when you're seated at the table. This way you'll do less unplanned snacking.

Keep your portions in control by not eating your favorite snack straight from the box or bag. Break snack down into one serving, and eat only that one serving.

Save some calories for snacks between meals.

Hate to waste food, put leftovers in a sealed zip bag or container and save for another meal.

Stay hydrated, dehydration can also make you feel sluggish and be mistaken for hunger. Be sure to drink throughout the day, and don't rely on thirst to remind you to have a glass of water. The average person needs an average of 8 glasses of water a day.

Drink a big glass of water at the start of every meal to help you fill up. End every meal with a large glass of water.

Keep a food journal, it will keep you accountable.

Use small plates. Research shows that you'll eat less because you'll think you actually ate more.

Don't have a big lunch and a big dinner on the same day. If you overeat at one meal then cut back at the next.

It is recommended to avoid a lot of caffeine, refined carbohydrates (sugar), alcohol, salt, and other food additives especially in large amounts, this can decrease your metabolic efficiency. Eating large amount of (bad sugar) carbohydrates will lead to an energy rush, and then a big crash, which may lead to fatigue. Excess amount of salt can disrupt your fluid balance, changing your daily water needs, which will increase your health risk like high blood pressure.

Don't think about what you can eat, focus on what you can eat more of like lean meats, fruits, vegetables, whole grains, fish, legumes and nuts.

In addition to following a proper diet and increasing your daily activities, and adding regular exercise to your program will help keep your body working more effectively by maintaining your energy levels, and speeding up your metabolism which will burn more calories.

Here are a few steps to follow in getting started to create your own Weight Management and Smart Eating Program:

1. Put a Plan Together.

2. Eat Right.

3. Stay Active.

4. Design an Exercise Program.

5. Keep a Daily Food Diary.

Put a Plan Together

See your doctor before you start any diet or exercise program. Especially if you have any health or risk factors such as high blood pressure or high cholesterol or if you are on any type of medications. You can measure your risk factors as your diet progresses. You can purchase an inexpensive digital blood pressure cuff for your arm or wrist to measure your own blood pressure on a daily basis. This will also help you to track your blood pressure progress as you lose weight. You should also purchase an inexpensive digital weight scale to keep progressive track of your weight. Two other items that may be needed that helps in determining food calorie contents is an inexpensive digital food scale, measuring cups and spoons.

To determine your daily calorie needs, this is your BMR plus your daily activities will give you your daily calorie needs, which is your AMR.

You will need to determine four AMR daily calorie counts:

1. Your Current AMR daily calorie count.
2. Your High Diet AMR daily calorie count.
3. Your Target AMR daily calorie count.
4. Your Low Diet AMR daily calorie count.

Perform the following four steps to determine your four AMR daily calorie counts.

Step 1: To determine your current AMR daily calorie count which is the calories needed to maintain your current weight. This can be done by using my AMR Daily Calorie Chart in Chapter 4, Example 4-1 below in this book to determine how many calories you need each day to maintain your current weight. This will be your current AMR daily calorie count.

> Example: If your current weight is 240 pounds, using the AMR Daily Calorie Chart in Chapter 4, Example 4-1 below in this book, your Current AMR daily calorie count will be around 2,200 to 2,600 calories a day, depending on your activity level.

Step 2: To determine your High Diet AMR daily calorie count, this would be your daily calorie count for your diet. You can do this by reducing your Current AMR daily calorie count by 500 to 1,000 calories per day, to determine the amount of weight you would like to lose weekly. This will be your High Diet AMR daily calorie count.

> Example: Taking your Current AMR daily calorie count (in Step 1 use the lowest calories in that bracket) of 2,200 calories a day and subtract 500 calories, gives you a High Diet AMR daily calorie count of around 1,700 calories a day.

Step 3: To determine your Target AMR daily calorie count use my AMR Daily Calorie Chart in Chapter 4, Example 4-1 below in this book to determine how many calories you need each day to maintain the weight you should weigh, this will be your Target AMR daily calorie count.

> Example: If your Target weight is 200 pounds, using the AMR Daily Calorie Chart in Chapter 4, Example 4-1 below in this book, your Target AMR daily calorie count will be around 1,800 to 2,200 calories a day, depending on your activity level.

Step 4: To determine your Low AMR daily calorie count

take the Target AMR daily calorie count and subtract 500 calories, this will be your Low AMR daily calorie count.

> Example: Taking your Target AMR daily calorie count (in Step 3 use the lowest calories in that bracket) of 1,800 calories a day and subtract 500 calories, gives you a Low Diet AMR daily calorie count of 1,300 calories a day. Maintaining an AMR daily calorie count of no less than 1,300 calories, (which is your Low AMR daily calories), and no more than 1,700 calories, (which is your High Diet AMR daily calories a day), will help you to lose 1 pound a week. Adding more daily activities or exercise may allow you to add 200 to 400 calories to your High Diet AMR daily calories a day.

It is not recommended for health reasons to decrease your calorie intake 500 calories below your Target Weights Daily AMR, your body will think its experiencing bad time or starving and your metabolism and energy levels will fall, and you will burn fewer calories.

As you lose weight your calorie needs will decrease so re-adjust your High Diet AMR daily calories, by performing Step 1 and Step 2 until you reach your target weight. It's recommended to start slowly with just a small reduction in calories per day. This is a lifestyle change and not a crash diet. Cutting out too many calories in the beginning you may find the calorie restriction too difficult and give up on improving on your eating habits. Also you should focus on a slow and gradual weight loss about one pound per week (a reduction of 500 calories per day from your daily AMR) is recommended.

Example: 4-1 Active Metabolic Rate (AMR) Daily Calorie Chart

Weight	Sedentary Calories	Moderate Calories
110	990	1210
120	1080	1320
130	1170	1430
140	1260	1540
150	1350	1650
160	1440	1760
170	1530	1870
180	1620	1980
190	1710	2090
200	1800	2200
210	1890	2310
220	1980	2420
230	2070	2530
240	2160	2640
250	2250	2750
260	2340	2860
270	2430	2970
280	2520	3080
290	2610	3190
300	2700	3300
310	2790	3410
320	2880	3520
330	2970	3630
340	3060	3740
350	3150	3850
360	3240	3960
370	3330	4070
380	3420	4180
390	3510	4290
400	3600	4400
410	3690	4510
420	3780	4620
430	3870	4730

The AMR Daily Calorie Chart should only be used to provide a rough estimate on daily calories needed and is a guideline, there are other considerations that may add or deduct calories needed such as body frame, your muscle mass, daily activities and genetic factors.

Sedentary – Job is office work with no physical demand, or/and little or no exercise a day.

Moderate - Job requires limited physical demand, or/and you exercise 30 to 60 minutes a day or more.

Eat Right

Since you're trying to learn a weight management and smart eating habit program you need to make sure every calorie counts, there is not much room for calories in junk foods or high calorie snacks. While learning weight management and smart eating habits increase your intake of lean proteins, fruits and vegetables that are high in nutrients and fiber but generally low in calories. Choose lean protein sources containing low fats found in poultry, chicken, turkey, fish and seafood. Always fix these food items broiled, baked or grilled never fry in oil or deep fried, and removing the skin will take off 20 percent of the calories of these food items which is where most of the fat is. Fried foods contain high levels of saturated and Trans fats and are also higher in calories. Avoid fried foods unless made with healthier low fat oils and even then use limited amounts. If red meat is in your menu for the day, remember red meats are higher in calories because of the fat content, cut off as much of the fat as possible. Choose lean cuts of meat and skinless chicken and limit your diet in eating lunch meats, bacon and fatty sausage.

If you're on a vegetarian diet to get your protein include soybeans and other beans, soy milk drinks (calcium enriched), lentils, tofu, cereals, milk, yogurt, cheese and eggs can enhance sufficient protein intake.

Avoid foods which are high in sugars or fats which are high in calories such as soft drinks, fruit drinks, potato chips, corn/tortilla chips, cheese puffs, buttered popcorn, candies, jams, sauces, ice cream, breakfast cereals, donuts, cookies, cakes, pies, pastries, all desserts, some canned foods, pizzas with meat toppings. Avoid deep fried foods like chicken, fish, French fries and onion rings. Choose medium size low fat hamburgers avoid the bacon. Avoid large sizes of latte and Frappuccino coffees, and request nonfat milk and no whipped cream. You can eat moderate quantities of these foods, but for serious weight control, look for low calorie or sugar free. Just be sure to watch your portion sizes so you don't eat too much of those foods which would cause you to cut good calories out of your daily intake.

Try to plan your meals and snacks ahead of time. When you are grocery shopping, avoid buying junk food and high calorie snacks. If the junk food and high calorie snacks are not in your house, you won't eat or want them. Eat slowly and chew your food thoroughly, this will help you eat less. Drink plenty of fluids preferably water or your favorite diet drink, your body needs fluids, and this will help fill you up faster. Make sure that your higher percentage of fluid intake a day is water, cut down or cut out all diet drinks if possible. If you're looking for a way to cut calories and increase your water intake try to keep a bottle of water in arms reach. Many people mistake thirst for hunger, which leads to excessive snacking. Instead of reaching for a snack, drink some water first. Keeping a bottle of water around will also remind you to drink water. If you are a soda addict try to swap soda for water, even if you prefer diet soda. Diet sodas generally contain many additives that aren't good for you. Try swapping sodas for plain water, if you need a flavor squeeze some lemon to add flavor, or try carbonated water. If you like to indulge in flavored lattes or mochas regularly, you could be taking in over 300 calories in just one drink. If you can't do without your morning fix, consider switching to simple coffee with a low-calorie sweetener. It's okay to use artificial or non-nutritive sweeteners to reduce your calorie intake, but you need to focus on good foods and not sugar free junk foods. Make your meal contain fewer calories by cutting back on the fats and sugars.

<u>Review and recommended Cooking Tips to help develop smart eating habits:</u>

Select water packed tuna instead of oil packed. This will cut calories by a third.

Use nonstick spray to sauté food, or rub oil onto the pan with a paper towel for the lightest possible coating.

If you must have goodies around for your family or company, don't make or buy your favorite kind.

Try to invest in single serving containers and use them for leftovers.

Use a tiny spoon when sampling your cooking, and if you're doing it a lot, eat less for dinner. The little tastes you take while cooking can really add up extra calories.

Let your toast or baked potato slightly cool before buttering so it absorbs less butter.

Remember that small changes add up. You will lose

12 or so pounds in a year just by giving up butter on your toast.

Prepare slow to eat foods like hot soups, uncut lean meat, or whole fruits.

Always keep a container of cooked brown rice in the fridge for a quick low-fat addition to left overs.

Chew sugarless gum while you are cooking, this will help to keep you from nibbling.

Switch to mustard if possible, it has no fat, instead of using mayonnaise.

Shop the perimeter of the grocery store where most meats, fresh fruit, vegetables, chicken, fish, eggs and dairy are located. Enter into the interior store aisles only with a shopping list in hand and avoid buying junk food and high calorie snack foods.

Never fry your fish, poultry or other cuts of lean meat. Only broil, roast or grill them.

Don't serve family style at the table, serve plates from the stove, if people want seconds, let them serve themselves, they'll be less likely to want seconds.

Make stews and soups ahead of time and refrigerate. Excess fat will float to the top, making it easy to remove the fat before reheating and serving.

Give away temptation and party leftovers. After a dinner party, pack up the leftovers and give it to your departing guests.

Flavor your meals with fresh or dried herbs and spices, salsa, vinegar or lemon.

Plan ahead and have healthy food selections on hand. Not having healthy options on hand makes it too easy to resort to fast food or bad eating choices.

Review and recommended tips that will help you to satisfy your Cravings:

If you like munching while watching TV, take up a hobby, or get into the habit of doing something that will keep your hands busy.

Savor what you're eating, especially the first two bites, which are the most flavorful, then throw the rest in the trash or save the rest for another time. This trick will help you eat less, and you may decide that some treats are not worth the calories.

Carry apples, bananas, oranges or whole grain crackers with you so you'll always have a low calorie snack on hand if you get hungry between meals.

Cravings take about 20 minutes to go away. If you can distract yourself for that long, you probably will have it beat.

Brush your teeth or rinse with mouth wash when you have a craving. The clean taste may dampen you craving.

When that favorite snack won't stop calling your name, close your eyes and visualize eating some. Chances are you'll eat less than usual or lose the craving.

If you're dying for chocolate, eat a couple bites, save the rest until later.

Eat what you're craving in its healthiest form, for example, instead of French fries go for a baked potato, if possible.

Eating at Home and throughout the Day

Don't load up your kitchen with tempting high calorie snacks, instead keep on hand fresh fruits, vegetables, whole grain crackers and a favorite cheese for snacking on. Never skip breakfast and for breakfast try to eat at least 300 calories containing plenty of protein and fiber. Eat fruits and vegetables between meals if possible which are low in calories and high in nutrients and fiber, this will keep you feeling full throughout the day. Try to break bad habits of eating while watching TV, but if this is hard to do, and you need a snack for this reason, measure out one serving of the snack you will be eating, don't take the whole bag of your snack item with you, this will tempt you into eating the whole bag. Drink a glass of water before having any snack or meal. Also remember one half cup of rice or pasta has about 100 calories, while one half cup of vegetables has only 14 calories. Try to eat 3 portion size meals a day, but as we age digestion slows, especially the digestion of fiber, so lightening the load by eating smaller, lighter meals and healthy snacks will keep your energy levels more stable and your metabolism up, so it's recommended to eat 5 small portion size meals a day that contains a variety of lean proteins, fruits and vegetables.

Eating at Fast Food and Restaurant Establishments

When going out to eat most Fast Food and Restaurant Establishments serve very large portions, unless you order the smaller. Eat at restaurants that either display or have available nutrition information that contains calorie information. If the restaurant serves large portions always ask for a take home box and take half of your meal home for another meal. Use portion control, instead of ordering a 12 or 16 oz. steak, order an 8 or 6 oz. This will save you from eating unnecessary calories. If you desire a steak for its thickness and must order the 12 or 16 oz. steak, cut it in half, take half home for another meal. If you are with a friend you can share with, split the meal and share it, not only will you save calories you would have eaten but also on the cost of the meal. You can also order from the appetizer menu for your main meal instead of an entrée. Another option is to order from the Children's menu or request the Lunch portion size for dinner, since the Children's menu and the Lunch menu portions are generally smaller.

No matter what type restaurant you're eating at, whether it's an American, Mexican, Italian, Chinese or any other restaurant type use the nutrition information provided to figure the calories per meal and use portion control to eat smarter.

Review and recommended Tips for Eating Right When Eating Out at Restaurants and Fast Food Establishments:

Drink a lot of water with every meal.

Always order a salad with your dressing on the side.

If French fries come with your order, ask for vegetables instead.

Only order a desert if you have a couple friends you can share it with.

At Fast Food Restaurants never supersize, and try to order the smallest calorie based sandwich, the bigger the sandwich the more calories it will contain.

If you order one of the bigger sandwiches, cut the sandwich in half, eat one half, and take the other half home for another meal.

Before going to a restaurant, check out its menu for a calorie count of the entrée you are going to order.

Wear fitted clothes or a slightly tight belt when dinning out. The feeling of restriction will send a stuffed signal to your brain.

When eating at a buffet or dinner party scope out everything that's available before eating. Save about a quarter of your plate for high calorie food and the rest for low calorie foods.

Have the bread basket or the free chips removed as soon as you sit down at a restaurant. The free bread or chips will add an addition 400 to 600 calories to your meal.

In a group if possible be the first to order so you won't be influenced by your friend's choices.

Be selective at a family gathering, skip the food you can get anywhere and only eat the special dishes if possible. You'll feel more than satisfied without inhaling hundreds of extra calories.

Order the simpler dishes, they're often less fattening because they don't contain any sauce.

Ask your waiter to keep your water glass filled, double the side of vegetables and cut the starches.

Eat a snack before going to a party, arriving with an empty stomach is a recipe for overeating.

At a restaurant eat only half your meal and take the rest home in a doggie bag to eat latter or the next day at another meal, or ask your partner to split a meal.

Portion Size and Control

With the free soda refills, supersized French fries, bread and chips at every restaurant establishment we are having trouble controlling how much we eat. But if you want to control your weight, you must practice portion control. A portion is the serving or amount of food. The actual serving size of any food you eat may be many times the portion amount suggested by the USDA guidelines, which means you may be eating more calories than you think and more than you need to maintain a proper weight. Researchers measured typical servings from takeout restaurants, fast food chains and family style eateries found that most foods served were many times the USDA recommended serving size. A portion is the amount of food or drink a person chooses to consume, but in most cases the portion eaten is larger than the serving size simply because most people don't know any better. Portion size and control is limiting what you eat and being aware of how much food you are actually eating and what calories are in that serving. With a little practice, portion control is easy to do and can help people to successfully reach and then maintain a proper weight.

At home for a couple of weeks you may have to measure and weigh all your food at first until you can recognize a portion by sight. Use measuring cups, spoons, and a food scale to measure out quantities of the food you eat. Also all packaged and canned food items bought at the grocery stores now contain nutrition labels on the product package that shows servings per package and the calories within, reference Appendix F, The Nutritional Fact Food Label. Just remember if the serving size is 2 and there are 200 calories per serving, the total calories in the packaged or canned item is 400 total calories. Cut down on the portion size of your meals you used to eat. Pay attention to nutrition labels and try to buy only foods in which 20 percent or fewer of the calories come from fat. This will automatically help control the amount of fat in your diet. Don't use "Low Fat" as an excuse to overeat. Just because a food says it's "Low Fat" doesn't mean you can eat double the amount. One portion is still one portion, even low-fat foods still contains calories.

When eating out at restaurants review the restaurants nutritional menu that contains the menu entrees which provides serving sizes and total calories per food item you can order. This will help you to figure out your total calories per meal when eating out at restaurants.

Its portion control as well as total calories in a portion of food that is eaten that counts, whether the calories come from carbohydrates, fats or proteins.

<u>Review and recommended Tips on Portion Size and Portion Control:</u>

Measure foods and beverages accurately using a measuring cup, tablespoon, teaspoon or food scale.

Learn how to estimate serving sizes by estimating portion sizes in comparison to known objects. For example three ounces of cooked meat, fish, or poultry is about the size of a deck of cards, one half cup serving is the size of an ice cream scoop, one cup serving is the size of a tennis ball, 1 ounce of cheese serving is the size of 4 dominos, and a medium potato is about the size of a computer mouse.

Measure your plates, bowls, cups and glassware in your kitchen to see what they actually hold. Always eat or drink from the smaller of these items.

Serve food from the stove instead of family style at the table, which discourages second helpings.

Premeasure food items into individual portions in zipper bags or sealed containers so when you are ready to eat or prepare that item you'll know the portion size and calorie count you're preparing instantly.

If you have an additive to put into your tea or coffee, put the additive into the cup before adding the beverage to better gauge the amount you used.

If eating out, in general, restaurant servings are considerably bigger than recommended portion sizes, only eat half or share the meal with a friend, or get a take home box and take the meal home and eat as another meal.

If eating a salad, order the dressing on the side, dip your fork into the dressing, then into your salad to conserve calories from the dressing.

Eat only when hungry and stop when satisfied or comfortably full.

Stay Active

Instead of lying around on the couch watching TV get out and do something, if it's only to go on a walk, you will burn calories and the extra activity will improve your mood and will distract you from your cravings. Sometimes this is hard to do after getting home from work, try to take as much advantage of the daylight as possible or throughout the day gardening, doing chores, walking, climbing stairs, and staying engaged and active. If you have a non-physical demanding job, park a distance from the front door so you have to walk further to your job. If there is an elevator, if possible take the stairs instead of the elevator. Try walking during your breaks and lunch period. Being more active during the day will improve your health and increase your AMR.

Design an Exercise Program

Increasing your physical activities and eating fewer calories is important for good health and weight loss, and will help you keep the weight off over time. If you have a non-physical demanding job or retired and you don't exercise now, think about joining a gym, or setting up a home workout plan for pushups, crunches, squats, jumping jacks, etc., you can also walk, jog or run when the weather is good. Sometimes this is hard to do after getting home from work. If time permits exercise before going to work, or include your exercise in your lunch period. People vary in the amount of physical exercise they need for weight control. Many can maintain or lose weight by exercising 30 minutes a day of moderate intensity exercise such as a brisk walk. Exercise will also benefit you by maintaining and improving your physical strength and fitness, and will help to manage and improve diseases like diabetes, heart disease and osteoporosis.

Review and recommended Workout and Motivation Tips to follow:

For better results for weight loss don't just diet, you also need to exercise which will help burn more calories, if it's only taking a 30 minute daily walk.

One of the best ways to rev up your metabolism is to do strength training exercises at least two to three times a week. Building muscle makes your body more efficient at burning fat throughout the day, even when you're resting. Also adding cardio in your workout enhances your health and fat burning, by doing strength training first and then followed up with a cardio workout, you will burn more calories.

Tape your favorite TV shows and watch them when you exercise.

Be sure to wear supportive sneakers and comfortable clothes so you feel good during your exercise period.

Get into a regular workout routine. You'll find out that as you get fit and healthy your appetite may change, especially the cravings for junk food.

Create a shorter walking route for days you're busy and pressed for time. It's better to do a short exercise routine than doing nothing at all.

Short bout of exercise each day is more effective than longer less frequent ones.

If possible work out first thing in the morning. This

will also give you more energy throughout the day, and your workout is done no matter how busy your day gets.

Exercising in a group or with friends will make a workout less dreary and you're more likely to stick to it.

Set small goals and as you reach each of them, reward yourself to something, whatever appeals to you.

Use a radio and turn up the music with a fast beat while you work out, it will help your workout and make time fly.

Instead of thinking you deserve to eat something, think that you deserve to be healthy and happy because you will look better by exercising instead of eating.

Have a calendar available in a prominent spot and mark your workout days and eating schedule. Being able to see the evidence of your hard work will inspire you to keep it up.

Keep a Daily Food Diary

You will increase your chances of success if you keep track of all the foods you eat during the day. Keeping track of the food and the calorie count of the foods you eat will help you stay on track when trying to lose weight or maintaining a desired weight and activity level. You can use a notebook or there are some online services that may be used. To help figure out the calories in your food items, you can purchase a good calorie counter book sold at most book stores, or there are some good services provided on line, you can also reference Appendix G,

Food Items Quick Calorie Reference in this book. Most foods and items sold in stores contain a nutritional label on them that explains serving size and the calorie count of the content, reference Appendix F, The Nutritional Fact Food label. Most restaurants provide a nutritional breakdown of their items provided and a breakdown of the items calorie count, also most chain restaurants also provide this information online. Don't let the diet industry brain wash you into thinking calorie counting or portion control is hard, so save your money on fad diets and spend it on something else.

Chapter 5

My Weight Management and Smart Eating Program

I took the following tools in this book and put a weight management and smart eating program together for myself. This is something I knew I needed to do, and something I knew I must do the rest of my life if I want to maintain a desired weight level. My goal was to lose 2 pound a week when I started out, and I knew it would take me two or more years to reach my goal, since I had 200 plus pounds to lose. I followed the following 5 steps and put together a plan that I could work with:

1. I started by putting a plan together that defined what I needed to do to accomplish my goals.
2. With regard to eating right I defined what I could and could not eat, which included portion control and calories needed to get my weight in control and maintain it.
3. I examined my activity level I was doing throughout the day and modified it to add more activity involvement to raise my AMR.
4. I put together an exercise program that fit my needs to improve my overall health and fitness even though this was optional.

5. I put together a daily food diary to track what I was eating throughout the day so I could track my calorie intake.

<u>My Plan Included</u>

I saw a doctor that cleared me to start a diet and exercise program. Even though my blood pressure was 155/115 which is considered high, my cholesterol levels were normal. I purchased an inexpensive digital blood pressure cuff that fits around the wrist so I could keep track of my blood pressure on a daily basis as my weight management program progressed. I also purchased an inexpensive digital weight scale to keep progressive track of my weight. Two other items that I purchased to determining food calorie contents is an inexpensive digital food scale, and a set of measuring cups and spoons. I also went to a book store and purchased a book that contained food items and their calorie counts to use for items I don't eat on a regular basis, this provided me a tool to obtain the calorie count of those items I needed.

By using the Height and Weight Chart in Chapter 3, Example 3-2, since I am 5' 9" it determined my weight should be around 167 pounds, but I have a large body frame so I added 20 pounds which put my desired weight at around 187 pounds. I set my target weight at 200 pounds. My current weight was 425 pounds, so I knew I had to lose at least 225 pounds. When I started my smart eating plan my weight was 425 plus pounds, and my AMR daily calorie intake was around 3,900 plus calories a day.

I determine my Current AMR daily calorie count since my current weight was 425 pounds, using the AMR Daily Calorie Chart in Chapter 4, Example 4-1 in this book, would be around 3,900 plus calories a day.

I set my High Diet AMR daily calorie count to 3,000 calories a day. I did this by reducing my Current AMR daily calorie count by 1,000 calories per day, hoping I could lose 2 pounds a week.

I set my Target AMR daily calorie count to 2,000 calories a day by using my AMR Daily Calorie Chart in Chapter 4, Example 4-1 in this book to determine how many calories I needed each day to maintain a weight of 200 pounds.

To stay within 500 calories of my Target AMR daily calorie count I set my Lowest Diet AMR daily calorie count to be above 1,500 calories a day. Keeping my weight management diet AMR daily calorie intake to be at least 1,500 calories a day and less than 3,000 calories a day, in the beginning I was able to lose 2 pounds a week. As I lost weight I re-adjusted my High Diet AMR daily calories until I reached my target weight, see the example below.

<u>My AMR Daily Calorie History from Start to End as it Pertained to my Weight Management Program</u>

Current Weight	Current AMR Daily Calories	High Diet AMR Daily Calories
425	4200	3000
400	4000	3000
375	3800	2800
350	3500	2500
325	3300	2300
300	3000	2000
275	2800	1800
250	2500	2000
225	2300	1800
200	2000	1500

Target AMR Daily Calories	Lowest Diet AMR Daily Calories
2000	1500
2000	1500
2000	1500
2000	1500
2000	1500
2000	1500
2000	1500
2000	1500
2000	1500
2000	1500

This is a short history of my AMR Daily Calorie requirements as it pertained to my weight at the start of my Weight Management Program of 425 pounds until I got my weight down to my target weight of 200 pounds. Because of my excessive weight, I was able to subtract 1,000 calories a day from my Current AMR daily calories which allowed me to lose 2 pounds a week in the beginning. If you only need to lose 40 or so pounds to get to your target weight, it's only recommended to subtract only 500 calories from your Current AMR daily calories which will allow you to lose 1 pound or so a week.

Eating Right

This section was hard for me to do. I loved food and if I only ate what they told me I could eat I knew I wouldn't last on this program and would go back to bad and uncontrolled eating habits. So I had to learn calorie counting and portion control. This is an easy process since most foods sold in grocery stores and chain restaurants provide nutrition information that gives you portion sizes and calorie counts per item. After a couple of weeks I was able to recognize by eye calorie counts per food items and proper portion servings. To start I set my daily calorie intake to be less than 3,000 calories a day, which allowed me to lose 1 to 2 pounds a week, which is a safe weight loss. I ate whatever I wanted throughout the day, keeping track of what I ate, and when I hit that magic number of 3,000 calories I was done eating for the day. I always tried to eat more than 1,500 calories a day and less than 3,000 calories a day when I started. I never gorged or ate my total days calories all at one time. I never skipped breakfast, and ate between 300 and 500 calories in the morning which sometimes included eggs, sausage and cheese. If I ate cereal I would eat no more than one serving and would use only 1% milk on my cereal. I never ate a traditional breakfast every morning, if there was pizza left over from the previous day, I'd have a slice of pizza, the left over half of a sub or sandwich, no matter what I had for breakfast I tried to limit it to around 300 calories. For the evening meal I saved at least 300 calories which left the balk of my calories to be eaten throughout the day. To help control my eating habits, I would only eat between 6 am and 6 pm, this helped me to cut out a lot of the after hour snacking. Since I was trying to learn a weight management and smart eating habit program I knew I needed to make sure every calorie counted, there was no way for me to avoid junk food or high calorie snacks, but I limited myself to small servings just to take care of the cravings I had for them. Throughout the day I would eat a variety of different food choices and tried to portion meals out to at least three meals a day or five small meals a day to include lean red meats, chicken, turkey, fish, seafood items, fruits and vegetables. I always tried to grill, broil or steam these food items. If made available I wasn't going to turn down any fried chicken or fish, but I would remove the skin, which is where most of the fat is, this helped me to save 20 percent of the calorie count of these items. If steak was on my menu for the day I'd cut off as much of the fat as possible to save on calories, for hamburgers I'd purchase the lean package of hamburger meat with the least percentage of fat. From time to time I would eat a sandwich or sub for lunch that included different lunch meats or even a hotdog, but I just kept track of the calorie count of the sandwich on my daily calorie count diary.

This was another area I knew I wasn't going to be able to do is avoid these food items the rest of my life fruit drinks, potato chips, corn/tortilla chips, cheese puffs, buttered popcorn, candies, jams, sauces, ice cream, breakfast cereals, donuts, cookies, cakes, pies, pastries, all desserts, some canned foods, pizzas with meat toppings, deep fried foods like chicken, fish, French fries and onion rings, which was recommended. All of these food items I knew are high in sugar, fat and calories, so I would limit myself to a small moderate portion of these items from time to time, and track them on my daily calorie count diary. Sometimes I'd just take a couple bites of the high calorie snack items I'd be craving and then throw the rest in the trash or pack it away and save for another time. This helped me to eat less of those bad items, but also satisfied my cravings. I knew if I ate too much of those food items it would cause me to cut good calories out of my daily calorie intake or cause me to consume too many calories for the day.

I got rid of all the snacks and junk foods in my house, and I didn't miss them, this also helped me to control my eating habit. I tried to plan my meals in advance, sometimes this would change throughout the day, and I would just make modification to my eating plans and adjust my calories per meals. When I first started my weight management program I was drinking 6 to 8 sugar sodas a day. I had to experiment but I was able to find a diet soda I could enjoy. Diet sodas are high in sodium and bad chemicals but I needed a fluid at the time to lower my daily calorie count. After a few months I started drinking bottled water and what I liked even better was the flavored carbonated water which helped me to replaced 50 percent of my fluid intake to water. I made my meals to contain fewer calories by cutting back on the items that contained high fats and sugars per meal.

At Home and throughout the Day

It was hard but I cut out all the in between meal snacks. I tried to preschedule my daily meals and would plan 3 portion size meals a day or 5 small portion size meals a day that included a variety of proteins, (good non-sugar) carbohydrates and limited my fat intake which kept me feeling full throughout the day. I would eat breakfast between 6 am and 8 am. I would have a mid-morning snack around 10 am, and then I'd eat a light lunch around 1 pm. I would have another mid-day snack around or late afternoon light lunch around 3 pm, and then my final meal for the day I would eat around 6 pm. I also only ate between the hours of 6 am and 6 pm to help control my eating habit. For special events and parties I would adjust my eating time when I had to eat after 6 pm.

Fast Food and Restaurant Establishments

I knew going out to eat at fast food and regular restaurant establishments they would serve large portions of food I would order and also high calorie. It was nothing for me at lunch at a fast food restaurant to consume at least a 1,700 or more calorie meal. Eating lunch or dinner at a regular restaurant it was easy for me to consume at least a 2,300 or more calorie meal. I would eat out 3 to 5 days a week. With a basic daily AMR of 2,000 calories a day to maintain a weight of 200 pounds there wasn't much room for all the other things I could eat throughout the day without overeating to include breakfast and a late night meal. So consuming 4,000 plus calories a day and maintaining a weight of more than 425 pounds was easy, because of my bad eating habits and the bad choices I made in eating.

I knew I couldn't avoid the rest of my life from eating out at fast food establishments so I had to learn to be able to cut calories so I wouldn't consume as many calories in one meal. I never supersize and I stopped ordering fries at all fast food establishments this saved me 300 to 400 calories per meal. I would take my double hamburger sandwich with cheese which by the restaurant nutrition information is 800 calories. I would cut that sandwich in half which would give me 2 sandwiches of 400 calories each. I would eat one half of the sandwich and take the other as a carryout to eat later or the next day at another meal. This would save me an extra 400 calories on my meal. If I was going to exceed my calories for the day, I could cut out the extras and order a diet soda and save another 500 calories. If ordering fried chicken,

I would order the 2 piece instead of the 3 piece and removing the skin would save an extra 20 percent of the calories. I always checked the restaurants nutrition information online before going or got a copy of the nutritional information at the fast food establishment I was at and used this strategy whether ordering hamburgers, chicken, fish, tacos and sub sandwiches or any entrée at all fast food restaurants. I knew what I was eating, the calorie content and cut down on my portion servings, which helped me to save calories per meal.

I always tried to eat at regular restaurants that provided nutrition information on the food items they provided at their establishment. I found most restaurants provide this information online, or I would get a copy of the nutritional information at the restaurant I was at. If I ordered a meal I knew was a large portion with a lot of calories, I always ask for a take home box and would take half of my meal home for another meal. I used portion control to help me control the calories consumed, instead of ordering a 12 or 16 oz. steak, I would order an 8 or 6 oz. steak. I could still enjoy going out to eat but this helped me to save from eating unnecessary calories at one visit. Sometimes I would only order from the appetizer menu for my main meal instead of an entrée, or I would order from the children's menu or request the lunch portion size for dinner, since the children's menu and the lunch menu portions are generally smaller. When the complimentary bread or chips are bought to my table, I limited myself to a moderate serving instead of over indulging like I would have done in the past. If I was ordering a full meal, I'd never order an appetizer. Most appetizers can range between 500 to 1,000 calories per appetizer, so unless there were 2 or 3 other people in my party to share it with, I would pass on the appetizer. If my meal came with side orders, I'd order a baked potato with a little butter or the steamed vegetables and a salad with the dressing on the side. I would only order a desert if I had a couple of friend to share it with, most deserts at restaurants can range from 800 to 1,200 calories. I always checked the restaurants nutrition information and use this strategy no matter what I would order from the menu at whatever restaurants whether it was an American, Chinese, Italian or Mexican or any restaurant establishment I visited. I always knew what I was eating, the calorie content and cutting down on my portion servings, helped me to save calories per meal.

Before my weight management program I would go to the buffet at least once and sometimes twice a week. And at the buffet I would go through the line 3 or more times. I stopped going altogether, but sometime in a group or a party I had no choice but learn how to eat at a place that had unlimited food available. I would only go through the buffet line once, which I estimated a plate to contain around 1,000 calories, depending on what I put on my plate. I would also have only one small serving of a desert.

Getting or Staying Active

With my weight problem I knew in order to get it under control I had to cut my calorie intake. Because I loved to eat, and in order to be able to eat a little more as I cut my calorie intake, I had to increase my activity level. I designed an exercise program for myself to do three days a week. The days I didn't exercise I'd go for a walk for about 30 minutes or so. For lunch I'd eat a light lunch and walk the rest of my lunch period. I started cutting my own grass instead of paying someone to cut it for me. Yard work is a great exercise for increasing your AMR daily calories. When shopping or going to the mall, I parked a distance so I had to walk further to the stores. If there were elevators or escalators, I would take the stairs. Being more active during the day helped me to improve my health by helping me to lose weight, and to increase my AMR, which also allowed me to eat more.

Design an Exercise Program

Choosing an exercising program was optional and being 58 years old this is something I wanted to do but knew age was against me, and in the past I loved my weight training program. Being supper over weight and out of shape I started walking three days a week, starting at one third a mile a day. I increased this as I went along, now I'm running 5 miles a day, three days a week. I saw a study somewhere that implied doing strength training before your cardio workout burns more calories. Three days a week on Mondays, Wednesdays, and Fridays I do 1 hour of weight or strength training, then I do my cardio workout right after, which is running. I can't run on the machines because I get bored too fast, and quit to easy, so I do all my running outside. On Tuesdays and Thursdays I do a 1 mile walk or run. I saved Saturday and Sunday for body rebuilding, so I don't exercise on those days. My weight or strength training program consists of three different routines. On Mondays my program consist of any routine that is a push exercise. Bench Press, Behind the Neck Presses, Dumbbell Presses for the Chest area, and Triceps Extensions, etc. On Wednesdays my program consist of any routine that is a pull exercise. Standup Curls, Lateral Pulls, Dumbbell Curls, Laterals Pulls on the Lateral Machine, Dead Lifts, Chin ups, and Lateral Pulls on the Chin up bar, etc. On Fridays my program consists of any routine that exercises the leg and stomach area. Squats, different stomach crunches, toe extensions. I found an outside 1 story stair fire escape accessible to me that I climb 10 stories once a week on my Friday workout, which is climbing the fire escape 10 times.

Your exercise program doesn't have to be as radical or as long as mine, a good 30 minute brisk walk a day is adequate.

Muscle vs. Fat: During your diet program while trying to lose weight and exercise, cutting calories from your daily diet, your body recognizes the shortage of calories or energy to maintain its current body functions at its current weight, so the body attacks the lean muscle mass and takes the protein from the muscles for the extra energy. Also when you get on the scales it may appear you didn't lose any weight, but what has happened mostly doing strength training, you may have lost 2 pounds of fat, but you may have also gained 2 pounds of lean muscle. This may happen until your body stabilizes. This is why it's important to get the proper amount of protein in your daily diet, for adults its 50g-120g a day, avoid crash diets, and eat the calories required not to exceed your High Diet AMR daily calorie intake. On a calorie reduction program eat from all the food groups but try to make the higher percent of your intake protein. But also expect to lose some strength until you get to your target weight, then eating normal at your target weight you will regain your lean muscle mass and strength back.

Keeping a Daily Food Diary

I increased my chances of success with the weight management program by keeping track in a daily diary all the foods I ate throughout the day and the calorie count of the foods. I used a note book and designed my own daily food diary. If a nutritional label wasn't available on a food item, I figured out the calories for that food item by using a good calorie counter book I purchased at a local book store, also Reference Appendix G, Food Items Quick Calorie Reference in this book. Shopping at the grocery store I would use the nutritional label information to figure out the serving size and the calorie count the food item had. When going out to dinner or lunch at a fast food establishment I used the nutritional information provided by the restaurants or the nutritional information online of the restaurant I was going to so I could see the calorie count of the food I was going to eat. Once I reached my desired weight, and got my weight management and eating habits under control I discontinue using my daily food diary. If I saw that I was starting to gain weight, I'd restart the daily food diary to evaluate what I was eating, which would help me get my weight management back under control.

Example: 5-1 Daily Food Diary
Month of September

Daily Calorie Count 2000

Date	Food Item	Calorie Count	Total Daily Calories	Calories Remaining for the Day
Mon 9 / 1	Breakfast	350	350	1,650
	Snack	100	450	1,550
	Lunch	800	1,250	750
	Snack	200	1,450	550

	Dinner	450	1,900	100
Tue 9 / 2	Breakfast	300	300	1700
	Snack	200	500	1,500
	Lunch	900	1,400	600
	Snack	200	1,600	400
	Dinner	400	2,000	0
Wed 9 / 3	Breakfast	250	250	1,750
	Snack	200	450	1,550
	Lunch	800	1,250	750
	Snack	100	1,350	650
	Dinner	600	1,950	50
Thur 9 / 4	Breakfast	300	300	1700
	Snack	200	500	1,500
	Lunch	900	1,400	600
	Snack	100	1,500	500
	Dinner	500	2,000	0

This is a sample of a Daily Food Diary I used, feel free to copy mine or design one that fits your needs.

Chapter 6

Conclusion

Avoid the fad diets and save your money, I tried a lot of them and they did not work for me. To lose weight and to keep it off, it's important to make life style changes with a focus on reducing calories from your food and beverages by cutting back on the fats and sugars and using portion control and increasing your activity levels throughout the day. A smart eating plan and portion control is the key to successful smart eating habits and a good weight management program. It doesn't matter what plan or diet you use to lose weight, the important part of any plan is the ability to learn smart eating habits and a weight management program to keep the weight off once you have lost it. Losing weight and keeping it off is a life change you have to continue the rest of your life, you can never return to your old bad eating habits. Remember there are four main parts to good weight management which are portion size, portion control, hydration and increasing your activity level. No matter what your age is there are three key elements of the fountain of youth which are proper diet, staying active and exercise, which overall will make you feel better and keep you healthier your whole life. Eat what you want, enjoy your food, but know what you are eating and the calories you are taking in. You have the choice of keeping a manageable weight, or practice uncontrollable eating habits and regret you're overweight.

Appendix A

Essential Vitamins and Nutrients needed every day during weight loss

Vitamin C: Vitamin C is crucial for boosting your immune system, helping wounds to heal, protecting against cancer, fighting against free radical damage and helps maintain healthy skin. Vitamin C also converts inactive folic acid into the active form and plays a role in the formation of hemoglobin, the protein that carries oxygen in red blood cells. Foods that contain vitamin C are broccoli, red bell peppers, cauliflowers, parsley, lemon juice, strawberries, romaine lettuce, tomatoes, kiwi, papaya, guava just about all fruits and vegetables contain some amount of vitamin C. You should get at least 200 mg daily.

Vitamin D: Vitamin D not only promotes bone health by aiding the body with absorbing calcium, and helping to build stronger bones and prevent bone loss, but is also a major factor in regulating your metabolism, taming hunger cravings, and boosting your immune system. With the help of calcium and magnesium, vitamin D will also improve cardiovascular health. The main source of vitamin D is exposure to sunrays. Foods that contain vitamin D are herring, salmon, halibut, cod liver oil, catfish, mackerel, oysters, sardines, tuna, shrimp, eggs, mushrooms and milk. It's recommended to take 2,000 IU daily.

Vitamin E: Vitamin E as an antioxidant protects our cells from free radicals, and may help protect against cancer and Alzheimer's disease. It is one of the four fat soluble vitamins that our body requires for optimal functioning. In a study it was found that persons over the age of 55 that took a combination of vitamin E, vitamin C, beta-carotene and zinc daily reduced their chances of developing macular degeneration, which leads to blindness, by 35 percent. Foods that contain Vitamin E are sunflower seeds, wheat germ, almonds, hazelnuts, peanuts, olive oil, spinach, broccoli, kiwifruit, mango and tomatoes. It's recommended to take 200 mg daily.

Calcium: Calcium is the largest mineral in our body, and partnered with vitamin D helps keep our bones in peak shape, as well as to maintain proper nerve function and healthy blood pressure. Calcium also plays a part in releasing hormones and enzymes that provide a wide array of biological functions. Calcium is also a mineral that works with vitamin D that helps you to shed fat. Calcium is stored in fat cells, and researchers think that the more calcium a fat cell has, the more fat the cell will release to be burned. Calcium also promotes weight loss by binding to fat in your GI tract, preventing some of it from getting absorbed into your bloodstream. Foods that contain calcium are dark leafy greens, oranges, sardines, broccoli, nuts, salmon, apricots, currants, tofu, figs, and low fat dairy products. If you diet doesn't include adequate amounts of calcium, it's recommended to take 2,500 mg of calcium daily.

Conjugated Linoleic Acid (CLA): CLAs are potent fat burners that are found, along with vitamin D and calcium, in dairy products. They are fatty acids that are created when bacteria ferments the food in the first part of the stomach of cows, sheep and other ruminant animals. The CLA that is created through fermentation then makes its way into the meat and milk of these animals. When we consume these foods, the CLA helps glucose enter body cells, so CLA can be burned for energy and not stored as fat. CLA also helps to promote fat burning, especially in muscles, where the bulk of our calorie burning takes place. CLA is found naturally in meat and dairy products.

Magnesium: Magnesium which is another bone builder, and also maintains blood circulation, supports cardiovascular health, and helps your muscles and nerves relax. Foods that contain Magnesium are nuts, Swiss chard, dark leafy greens, sunflower seeds, dark chocolate, squash, pumpkin, cucumbers, black beans, navy beans, cereals, and bran. Men should get about 420 mg daily, women 320 mg daily.

Omega 3 fatty acids: Omega 3 fatty acids are the building blocks of fats, which curbs inflammation, regulates blood clotting, build cell membranes and supports cell health. Omega 3 fatty acids boost brain health, improves muscle growth, fights inflammation and decreases stress. Omega 3 is a polyunsaturated fat, which contributes to peak cardiovascular health by reducing blood triglycerides and LDL cholesterol helping to cut the risk of heart attack, stroke or similar events. Omega 3 fatty acids enable weight loss by switching on enzymes that trigger fat burning in cells. Foods that contain Omega 3 are fatty fish like salmon, tuna, sardines, and mackerel, walnuts, flaxseeds, hempseeds, wild rice, and Omega 3 fortified dairy products and Omega 3 enriched eggs. Take nature made fish oil 300 mg daily.

Reference also: Appendix D, Foods that Help Fight Fat, Salmon

Appendix E, Best Foods to Eat While Dieting and Weight Loss, Salmon

Appendix B

Foods that Suppress Your Appetite and will also Keep You Fuller Longer

We all suffer from bad eating habits that can lead to eating snacks in between meals that are high in calories, sugar and fat that will leads to unexplained weight gains. While dieting instead of popping hunger suppressant pills that are supposed to suppress your hunger, eating can actually suppress your appetite as long as you choose the right foods. I've tried these foods and they work to keep your appetite in check.

Almonds: All nuts have heart healthy fats, but almonds contain the most fiber per serving, which will keep you fuller longer. Eating 1 serving or just a small handful of almonds between meals can stave off that energy dip, which will help you to avoid those high calorie snacks you would normally eat. One study showed that our bodies may not absorb all of the fat in almonds, which might lead to an overall lower calorie intake when eating them. Remember 1 serving size or 1 oz. is 170 calories, so eating too many almonds may contribute significant calories to your daily intake.

Reference Also: Appendix C, Foods that will Boost Your Immune System

Appendix E, Best Foods to Eat While Dieting and Weight Loss

Avocados: Avocados are filled with fiber and heart healthy monounsaturated fat, which might be the perfect fill you up food. Foods high in fiber and rich in fat take longer to digest, allowing you to experience less overall hunger and possibly eat fewer calories. Avocados contain oleic acid which is a monounsaturated fat that tells your brain that your stomach is full.

Reference Also: Appendix D, Foods that Help Fight Fat

Appendix E, Best Foods to Eat While Dieting and Weight Loss

Cayenne Pepper: Cayenne Pepper spice is a proven appetite suppressant, and research found that people who added half a teaspoon of the red pepper to a meal ate 60 fewer calories during their meal. Half a teaspoon of cayenne pepper over some food can cause your body to burn an additional 10 calories.

Eggs: A recent study found that people who ate eggs for breakfast took longer to get hungry later. The participants had lower levels of ghrelin, which is an appetite stimulating hormone that tells the brain to eat, and higher levels of PPY, a hormone that helps stomachs feel full longer. Eggs are a perfect combination of protein and fat, which makes them more satisfying than any other breakfast food. If you're worried about the cholesterol because of the high content in the egg yolk, eggs aren't the main culprit in raising blood cholesterol. If there's a cholesterol concern or problem try just eating the egg whites, which also contain protein which will help keep you fuller longer.

Reference Also: Appendix E, Best Foods to Eat While Dieting and Weight Loss

Greek Yogurt: Greek yogurt is high in calcium and low in sugar, and is protein packed. A six ounce serving contains 15 to 20 grams of protein which is twice the amount in regular yogurt and the same as in a piece of lean meat. The protein in this food is one of the main factors in feeling full longer.

Reference also:	Appendix C, Foods that will Boost Your Immune System, Yogurt
	Appendix D, Foods that Help Fight Fat, Yogurt

Legumes: A serving of beans, lentils, chickpeas or even peanuts delivers the right lean protein, complex carbohydrates and good fats that can keep blood sugars stable which means getting a full feeling longer and keeping it.

Soup: Soup eaters experienced fewer craving throughout the day. The soups high water content along with the fiber filled vegetables and the hot temperature is the reason for the full feeling which will curb your appetite. Try to avoid creamy soups which can be fatty and high in calories.

Water: Water is critical for keeping organs, joints, tissues and the digestive system functioning well, and water also curbs hunger. Drink water anytime you feel hungry. People who drink a class of water before a meal will eat less than persons that drink no water.

Appendix C

Foods that will Boost Your Immune System

While on a diet or anytime eat these foods that will help boost your immune system and keep it running strong. Throughout my diet and even now I eat these food items.

Almonds: Almonds contain vitamin E which is also a key to a healthy immune system. Vitamin E is a fat soluble vitamin, meaning it requires the presence of fat to be absorbed properly. Nuts especially almonds are packed with vitamin E. A half cup serving will provide 100% of the daily recommended amount.

Reference also: Appendix B, Foods that Suppress Your Appetite and will also Keep You Fuller Longer

Appendix E, Best Foods to Eat While Dieting and Weight Loss

Broccoli: Broccoli is super charged with an arsenal of vitamins and minerals ready to do battle with any germ or infection, packed with vitamins A, C, and E, as well as numerous antioxidants. Broccoli is one of the healthiest vegetables you can eat. The key to keeping its power intact is to cook as little as possible, or better yet eat it raw.

Reference also: Appendix E, Best Foods to Eat While Dieting and Weight Loss

Citrus: Citrus tops the type of foods that keep our immune system running at 100%. Vitamin C in Citrus helps increase the production of white blood cells, which are a key to fighting infections. Because your body doesn't produce or store it, daily intake of Vitamin C is essential for continued health.

Reference also: Appendix E, Best Foods to eat While Dieting and Weight Loss, Grapefruit, Oranges

Garlic: Garlic was recognized early on for fighting infections and modern medicine has shown that garlic helps lower cholesterol and prevents hardening of the arteries. Its immune boosting properties come from a heavy concentration of allicin which is the principle biological active compound of garlic.

Ginger: Ginger is like vitamin C and can also help prevent colds. While it's used in many sweet desserts, ginger packs some heat in the form of gingerol, a relative of capsaicin, which gives chili peppers their distinctive heat. It's said ginger may possess cholesterol lowering properties.

Green Tea: Green Teas are packed with flavonoids, which is a type of antioxidant. Green tea also contains high levels of epigallocatechin gallate, or EGCG, which is another antioxidant. Green tea is also a good source of the amino acid L-theanine, which aids in the production of germ fighting compounds in your T-cells.

Reference also: Appendix D, Foods that Help Fight Fat

Appendix E, Best Foods to eat While Dieting and Weight Loss

Red Bell Peppers: Red Bell Peppers ounce for ounce has twice as much vitamin C, as well as being a rich source of beta carotenes, which are fat-soluble unsaturated hydrocarbons that can be converted into vitamin A in the body, than citrus fruits.

Spinach: Spinach is rich in vitamin C and also contains numerous antioxidants and beta carotene, which have been proven to increase the infection fighting cells of our immune system. Similar to broccoli, it's best cooked as little as possible or raw so that the nutrients are retained.

Turmeric: Turmeric is a key ingredient in many curries and has been used for years as an anti-inflammatory in treating osteoarthritis and rheumatoid arthritis. Turmeric has been shown to contain strong flu and cold fighting properties.

Yogurt: Yogurt selecting, select the yogurts that have "Live and Active Cultures" printed on the label and brands fortified with vitamin D. Recent studies suggest these cultures help stimulate your immune system to help fight diseases.

Reference also: Appendix B, Foods that Suppress Your Appetite and will also Keep You Fuller Longer, Greek Yogurt

Appendix D, Foods that Help Fight Fat

Appendix D

Foods that Help Fight Fat

Whole unrefined foods are great because your metabolism has to work harder to break them down than processed ones, so you're burning more calories and storing less fat. Try some of these fat burners, they worked for me.

Avocado: Avocado's unique combination of essential fatty acids, monounsaturated fats and antioxidant keeps inflammation in check and blood vessels clear and supple for a speedy metabolism.

Reference also: Appendix B, Food that Suppress Your Appetite and will also Keep You Fuller Longer

Appendix E, Best Foods to Eat While Dieting and Weight Loss

Beans: Beans are high in resistant starch and fiber that forces your system to (use extra energy) burn more calories to break them down.

Reference also: Appendix E, Best Foods to Eat While Dieting and Weight Loss

Coffee: Coffee contains caffeine that temporarily perks up your metabolism by as much as 15%. Caffeine also helps mobilize the forces that burn stored fat.

Chili Peppers: Chili Peppers "chilies" the heat signals the presence of capsaicin, a compound that along with capsiate, can propel the body to burn an extra 50 to 100 calories a spicy meal.

Green Tea: Green tea contains caffeine and antioxidants called catechin, believed to stimulate your nervous system and increase fat burning.

Reference also: Appendix C, Foods that will Boost Your Immune System

Appendix E, Best Foods to Eat While Dieting and Weight Loss

Salmon: Omega-3s in salmon and other fatty fish help build muscle, and the muscle you have, the more calories you burn. Omega-3s may also help reduce fat storage by lowering cortisol levels.

Reference also: Appendix A, Essential Vitamins and Nutrients Needed Every Day during Weight Loss, Omega 3 fatty acids

Appendix E, Best Foods to Eat While Dieting and Weight Loss

Yogurt: Yogurt has up to 50% more calcium per ounce than milk and contains probiotics that may keep belly fat under control. Calcium rich foods have slimming superpowers.

Reference also: Appendix B, Foods that Suppress Your Appetite and will also Keep You Fuller Longer, Greek Yogurt

Appendix C, Foods that will Boost Your Immune System

Appendix E

Best Foods to Eat while Dieting and Weight Loss

These foods are very nutritional that helps build bones, prevents chronic disease, and even keeps your mind sharp. New evidence from research suggests these foods can also help you to lose weight and keep it off. I ate these during my weight loss period and still enjoy them today.

Almonds are rich in healthy fats that help you slim down. For a snack, eat a handful of almonds instead of a high sugar calorie snack.

Reference also: Appendix B, Foods that Suppress Your Appetite and will also Keep You Fuller Longer

Appendix C, Foods that will Boost Your Immune System

Avocados contain oleic acid, a compound which is a healthy monounsaturated fat may trigger your body to kill hunger. Eat one half of an avocado daily, this will also melt belly fat. The creamy fruit is also packed with fiber and protein.

Reference also: Appendix B, Foods that Suppress Your Appetite and will also Keep You Fuller Longer

Appendix D, Foods that Help Fight Fat

Bananas contain resistant starch. A slightly green medium size banana will fill you up and boost your metabolism with its 12.5 grams of resistant starch. A ripe banana still ranks high on the list of foods containing resistant starch with about 5 grams.

Black beans, a cup of these beans are packed with about 15 grams of protein and doesn't contain any of the saturated fat found in other protein sources, like red meat.

Reference also: Appendix D, Foods that Help Fight Fat, Beans

Blueberries are known for their anti-aging effects. One cup of blueberries contains only 80 calories with 4 grams of fiber, and will help you feel full.

Broccoli cooked or raw is well known for its cancer preventing power and help control weight problems. One serving of broccoli is high fiber and is less than 30 calories.

Reference also: Appendix C, Foods that will Boost Your Immune System

Brown rice is high in fiber. A half cup serving contains 1.7 grams of resistant starch, a healthy carbohydrate that boosts your metabolism and burns fat. Brown rice is a low energy density food, that's very filling but low in calories.

Cheese (goat cheese) and feta contain a fatty acid that helps you feel full and burn more calories. Look for cheeses labeled (grass fed), those will have the highest content of this healthy fat.

Dark chocolate can slow down digestion so you feel full longer and eat less at your next meal. Dark chocolate is full of MUFAs, and studies show that eating a diet high in these healthy fats can speed up your metabolism to burn fat and calories. It may also curb cravings for salt, sweets, or fatty calorie wreakers.

Eggs get a bad rap when it comes to weight loss. But for breakfast the egg is loaded with protein that will curb your appetite. A study found that egg eater's don't have higher levels of bad cholesterol or lower levels of good cholesterol than bagel eaters.

Reference also: Appendix B, Foods that Suppress Your Appetite and will also Keep You Fuller Longer

Garbanzo beans or known as chickpeas, are packed with more than 2 grams of resistant starch per a half cup serving. They're also a great source of fiber, protein and healthy fats.

Grapefruit, eating half a grapefruit before each meal may help you to lose up to a pound a week. Grapefruit can lower insulin, a fat storage hormone, which may lead to weight loss. It's also a great source of protein, and being 90% water can feel you up so you will eat less.

Reference also: Appendix C, Foods that will Boost Your Immune System, Citrus

Green tea hydrates like water, which can help you feel up and eat less, and help shed pounds. The antioxidants in green tea will speed up your fat and calorie burn.

Reference also: Appendix C, Foods that will Boost Your Immune System

Appendix D, Foods that Help Fight Fat

Kidney beans, or red beans as they are known, offers protein and fiber, more than 5 grams per serving. One half cup serving of kidney beans contains about 2 grams of resistant starch.

Lentils are a great source of satiating protein and fiber. One serving, a half cup has 3.4 grams of resistant starch, which is a healthy carbohydrate that boosts metabolism and burns fat.

Low fat milk contains fatty acid, proteins and calcium which will keep you feeling satisfied and full.

Oats are rich in fiber, so a serving can help you feel full throughout the day. A half cup of oats contains 4.6 grams of resistant starch, a healthy carbohydrate that boost metabolism and burns fat.

Oranges are about 59 calories and contain a high amount of fiber, which will help you feel full and eat less throughout the day.

Reference also: Appendix C, Foods that will Boost Your Immune System

Pearl barley as a starchy side makes a slimming complement to a low calorie meal by adding fiber, and a half cup serving contains 2 grams of resistant starch.

Pears are a great snack, and one pear will contain 15% of your daily recommended fiber. Eat the pear un-peeled, the skin is where all the fiber is.

Pine nuts are packed with the same healthy fatty acids as almonds that will quell hunger hormones and burns belly fat. Approximately 80 nuts only contain 95 calories.

Plantains, a half cup of plantains contain almost 3 grams of resistant starch, a healthy carbohydrate that boosts metabolism and burns fat.

Potatoes are high in carbohydrates but are three times as filling as a slice of white bread and contain the same satiety index as oranges. Potatoes are high in resistant starch which helps your body burn fat.

Quinoa is another diet friendly whole grain. Quinoa is high in hunger fighting protein which will help you stay full longer on fewer calories and will help you to avoid overeating at other meals.

Salmon contains lean sources of protein and is a leaner choice than red meat, which helps you feel full without adding fat.

Reference also: Appendix A, Essential Vitamins and Nutrients Needed Every Day during Weight Loss, Omega 3 Fatty Acid

Appendix D, Foods that Help Fight Fat

White beans, a one half cup serving is high in fiber and contains approximately 4 grams of resistant starch that will helps to boost your metabolism.

Wine contains resveratrol, an antioxidant found in grape skin, which stops fat storage. Drinking a glass of wine can increase your calorie burn for a good 90 minutes.

Appendix F

The Nutritional Fact Food Label

The Nutritional Fact Food Label is required on all packaged food products in the United States. Most restaurants also provides online or at the establishment a Nutritional Fact Food breakdown of the items provided on their menu containing valuable information for people interested in eating smarter and healthier. Below are some of the facts and information that's provided on the Nutrition Fact Food Labels.

Serving size is the number of servings per packaged food item and the calories the serving contains. If the packaged food item contains 2 servings and each serving contain 100 calories, if you ate the whole packaged item you would consume 200 calories. So pay close attention to a packaged food item serving size and calories per serving.

Calories and Calories from Fat is an important number if you want to lose weight. You need to burn more calories than you eat daily. You also need to keep the calories from fat you eat each day below 35 percent of your total calories.

Fats are high calorie, so you need to choose foods that are lower in fat. The label also lists amount of saturated fat and Trans fats in each serving. You want to choose foods that are low in saturated and extremely low in Trans fats because they can raise your blood cholesterol and increase your risk of heart disease. On the other hand polyunsaturated and monounsaturated fats can help lower your cholesterol.

Cholesterol should be limited to less than 300 milligrams per day if you're healthy, else less than 200 milligrams per day if you have heart disease.

Sodium (salt) content can cause high blood pressure, so you should keep your daily sodium intake levels below 2,400 milligrams per day.

Carbohydrates that are on the food label lists the total carbohydrates and also shows the amount of carbohydrates that comes from either dietary fiber or sugar. Subtract the amount of fiber and sugar from the total carbohydrates to get an idea of how many complex carbohydrates are in each serving. Dietary fiber aids in your digestion and help lower your risk of heart disease and diabetes while increasing your feeling of fullness. Sugars on the other hand burn quickly and can raise your blood glucose levels.

Proteins burn slowly and are essential for building tissue and muscle. Look at the number of protein grams in each serving and the percentage of daily protein it provides.

Vitamins and minerals on the food label can help you determine if the food is high or low in certain vitamins and minerals, including calcium and iron. Each nutrient listed on the Nutrition Facts food label comes with a Daily Value (DV) percentage that shows you how much of the recommended daily allowance is contained in a single serving of that food product. Food products that are a good source for a particular vitamin contain 10 percent to 19 percent DV of that nutrient in each serving.

Review the Daily Value percentages because you need to eat a certain amount of unsaturated fats, carbohydrates, proteins, minerals and vitamins each day to stay healthy. You also need to limit your daily intake of unhealthy ingredients like saturated fats, Trans fats and sodium. Each nutrient listed on the Nutrition Facts food label comes with a percentage that shows you how much of the recommended daily allowance is contained in a single serving of that food item. If you see zeros there, you food won't have much nutritional value.

Appendix G

Food Items Quick Calorie Reference

Vegetables contain 25 calories and 5 grams of carbohydrate. One serving equals:

½ Cup	Cooked Vegetables
1 Cup	Raw Vegetables or Salad Greens
½ Cup	Vegetable Juice

Fruits contain 15 grams of carbohydrate and 60 calories. One serving equals:

1 Average	Apple, Banana, Orange, Nectarine, Peach, Kiwi
½	Grapefruit
½	Mango
1 Cup	Fresh Berries (Strawberries, Raspberries, Blueberries)
1 Cup	Melon cubes
1/8th	Honeydew melon
4 oz.	Unsweetened Juice
4 tsp.	Fruit Jelly or Jams

Starches contain 15 grams of carbohydrate and <u>80 calories</u> per serving. One Serving Equals:

1 Slice	Bread
2 Slices	Reduced Calorie or Lite Bread
¼ (1 oz.)	Bagel (Large)
½	English Muffin, Hamburger Bun
¾ Cup	Cold Cereal
1/3 Cup	Rice (Brown or White), Barley or Couscous, Legumes, (Dried Beans, Peas, Lentils), cooked
½ Cup	Pasta, Bulgar, Corn, Sweet Potato, Green Peas, cooked
3 oz.	Baked Sweet or White Potato
¾ oz.	Pretzels
3 Cups	Popcorn (Hot Air or Microwaved Popped)

Very Lean Protein contains <u>35 calories</u> and 1 gram of fat per serving. One serving equals:

1 oz.	Turkey Breast, Chicken Breast, skin removed
1 oz.	Fish Fillet, broiled
1 oz.	Canned Tuna in water
1 oz.	Shellfish (steamed/broiled)
¾ Cup	Cottage Cheese, Non-fat or Low Fat
2	Egg Whites
¼ Cup	Egg Substitute
1 oz.	Fat Free Cheese
½ Cup	Beans, cooked (black kidney, chick peas, lentils)

Lean Protein has 55 calories and 2 to 3 grams of fat per serving. One serving equals:

1 oz.	Chicken, Turkey (Dark Meat - Skin Removed)
1 oz.	Salmon, Swordfish, Herring, Lean Beef, Lean Chop of Veal, Lean Chop of Lamb, Pork Tenderloin or Fresh Ham
1 oz.	Low Fat Cheese
1 oz.	Low Fat Luncheon Meats
¼ Cup	4.5% Cottage Cheese
2 med.	Sardines

Medium Fat Proteins have 75 calories and 5 grams of fat per serving. One Serving Equals:

1 oz.	Beef, Corned Beef, Ground Beef, Pork Chop (With Fat Removed)
1	Medium Egg
1 oz.	Mozzarella Cheese
¼ Cup	Ricotta Cheese
4 oz.	Tofu

Fat Free and Very Low Fat Milk contain 90 calories per serving. One serving equals:

1 Cup	Milk, fat free or 1%
¾ Cup	Yogurt, plain nonfat or low fat
1 Cup	Yogurt, artificially sweetened

Fats contain 45 Calories and 5 grams of fat per serving. One Serving Equals:

1 tsp.	Oil (Vegetable, Corn, Canola, Olive), Butter, Stick Margarine, Mayonnaise
1 Tbsp.	(Reduced Fat Margarine, Mayonnaise), Salad Dressing, Cream Cheese
2 Tbsp.	Lite Cream Cheese
1/8	Avocado
8 Large	Black Olives
1 Slice	Bacon

www.ingramcontent.com/pod-product-compliance
Lightning Source LLC
Chambersburg PA
CBHW050420290526
45786CB00003B/1335

* 9 7 8 1 4 8 1 7 0 9 6 4 4 *